YOUR KNOWLEDGE HAS VALUE

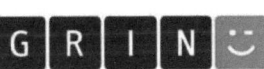

Natural Alternatives for Enamel Protection. Plant and Marine Extracts as Antimicrobial Solutions

Jemima Doreen Offei Agyepong

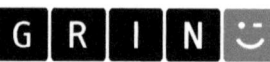

Bibliographic information published by the German National Library:

The German National Library lists this publication in the National Bibliography; detailed bibliographic data are available on the Internet at http://dnb.dnb.de.

ISBN: 9783346953162
This book is also available as an ebook.

© GRIN Publishing GmbH
Trappentreustraße 1
80339 München

Print and binding: Books on Demand GmbH, Norderstedt, Germany
Printed on acid-free paper from responsible sources.

The present work has been carefully prepared. Nevertheless, authors and publishers do not incur liability for the correctness of information, notes, links and advice as well as any printing errors.

GRIN web shop: https://www.grin.com/document/1399631

RESEARCH PROJECT

NATURAL ACTIVES IN ENAMEL PROTECTION: MARINE AND PLANTS EXTRACTS (LITERATURE REVIEW)

JEMIMA DOREEN OFFEI AGYEPONG

School of Pharmacy and Biomolecular Sciences, MSc Cosmetic Science, Liverpool John Moores University, United Kingdom

A dissertation submitted in partial fulfilment of the requirements for the degree of **MSc Cosmetic Science**

ABSTRACT

Objectives: Dental caries is one of the most common, costly, and prevalent oral diseases in the world. Caries is multifactorial and begins with the formation of dental biofilms on the enamel. Biofilms occur during the acid production of glucosyltransferase at low pH creating a viable environment for cariogenic bacteria to exist. To effectively inhibit the activities of cariogenic pathogens, preventive agents such as fluoride and chlorhexidine are mostly used. However, natural products may be alternative sources of caries prevention since they possess varieties of antimicrobial properties and provide minimal side effects as compared to the aforementioned. The aim of this literature review-based project is to explore biological active sources of marine and plant extracts that protect the enamel through their antimicrobial activity against cariogenic bacteria.

Methods: A comprehensive review was conducted on existing literature to search for publications on oral care and natural products and caries prevention. The databases of Google scholar, Science Direct, PubMed and Web of Science were searched for relevant and related articles using a combination of controlled vocabulary.

Results: Natural products were identified to possess different types of antimicrobial effect on cariogenic bacteria. The extracts were found to consist of bioactive compounds that inhibit the activities of dental biofilms, disrupt their adherence to the enamel, reduce demineralisation and promote stronger tooth structure. A summary of all the natural extracts, biological active compounds and their antimicrobial activity on oral microorganisms is presented in a tabular.

Conclusion: With the publications found on the related topic, it was evident that natural extracts from marine and plant sources exhibited antimicrobial activities that were effective against cariogenic bacteria and therefore alternative sources for caries prevention. However, there are challenges to overcome to optimise the effectiveness of natural extracts.

Key words: natural actives, dental caries, cariogenic bacteria, *Streptococcus mutans*, anti-caries, antimicrobial activity, bioactive compounds.

TABLE OF CONTENTS

List of Figures

List of Tables

"If you have teeth, Care!!!".

CHAPTER ONE: INTRODUCTION

1.1 Background

Oral hygiene is an essential part of human health. Maintaining good oral hygiene is one sure way of preventing dental caries, plaque, gingivitis, dental erosion, and mouth odour. Good oral hygiene also boosts an individual's self-esteem because it affects how they eat, chew, drink, socialise and enjoy life. Tackling oral diseases should be of great concern because it is associated with other chronic and public health diseases and as such its role in an individual's well-being coupled with its treatment mechanisms become expensive (Sheiham, 2005). In some extreme cases, people may lose all their teeth due to poor oral health (Selwitz et al., 2007) or suffer from discomfort and pain. The WHO (World Health Organisation) lists oral hygiene and dental caries as a worldwide public health threat especially in cases of children (Marinho et al., 2016). As a result of some of these undesirable reasons, oral hygiene should be tackled seriously with particular attention to the protection of the enamel which is the main organ in the mouth affected by oral pathogens.

Enamel, which is the white outer layer of the tooth is made up of calcium in the form of hydroxyapatite ($Ca_{10}(PO_4)_6(OH_2)$) (Li et al., 2014) and functions as a protection against internal and external pressures such as chewing, chipping, biting, sugar, cold and hot substances. The enamel also consists of 3% water and 1% organic matter made up of proteins and lipids. The average size of the enamel is about 50 nm wide by 25 nm thick and several microns long although size may vary with depth. (Jones, 2001).

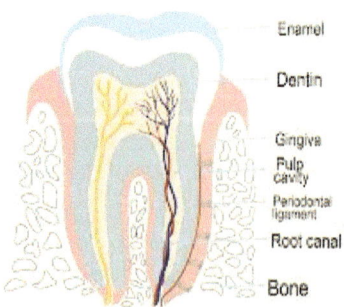

Figure 1 : shows diagram of the structure of the tooth adapted from dreamstime.com (Dreamstime.com, 2000-2021)

1.2 Dental caries effect on enamel

With the hardest outer layer of the enamel and its oral environment being surrounded by saliva, it is expected that the enamel would last a lifetime without its tissues being affected by erosion or caries. However, there are harsh factors which can rip off minerals from the enamel tissues (West and Joiner, 2014). Factors like the attack of bacteria from food and fizzy drinks deposit acid fermentation on the enamel which then forms plaque resulting in dental erosion and caries. Bacteria may break down sugars in the mouth and produce acids causing damage to the enamel and changes in colour, shape, function, sensitivity, and hardness to the tooth surface. (West and Joiner, 2014). This process is known as demineralisation (Martins et al., 2018) .Damage to the enamel may cause cavities below a pH of 5.5 (Li et al., 2014) leading to dental caries. Destruction of the enamel also affects the appearance, efficacy, and sensitivity of the tooth(Ferreira et al., 2013). Consuming high amount of sugar and inconsistent eating habits may contribute to the formation of bacteria in the mouth. It has been estimated that approximately 600 bacterial pathogens exist in the mouth (Bora et al., 2014), some of which are beneficial and the others being detrimental to the oral environment. Dating back to the Ancient Greeks, studies have linked the consumption of sugary commodities to damage of the enamel (Lutovac et al., 2017). In these studies, a relationship between the amount of sugar consumed and dental caries was established (Newbrun, 1982).

Dental caries also known as tooth decay is a multifactorial, microbiological largely occurring chronic diseases that affect people all over the world (Selwitz et al., 2007). Dental caries has been termed as a public health problem mainly among children (Fraihat et al., 2019) but can also affect adults. Caries formation begins when there is a collection of sticky complexes caused by pathogens. This is known as biofilms or dental plaque. Dental plaque is characterised by billions of bacteria found in the oral cavity by multi species biofilms(Selwitz et al., 2007, West and Joiner, 2014). Despite the numerous bacteria found in the oral cavity; the pathogens associated with dental caries are limited. These bacteria include *Lactobillus spp, Streptococcus mutans (S. mutans), Streptococcus sobrinus (S. sobrinus), Streptococcus salivarius (S. salivarius)* and *Actinomyces spp* (Deo and Deshmukh, 2019). However, the main aetiological factor of dental caries is *Streptococcus mutans* which is a gram-positive bacterium with the ability to withstand acidic conditions on the tooth surface (Kleinberg, 2002).

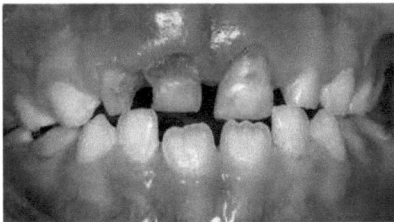

Figure 2: Shows a picture of dental caries adopted from www.nature.com (Morgan, 2008)

The process of dental caries can be controlled by numerous factors such as salivary flow and the use of fluoride and chlorhexidine found in toothpastes and mouthwashes. Saliva plays an important role in protecting the oral tissues. The presence of its organic and inorganic compounds exhibit antimicrobial effect against dental caries (Lenander-Lumikari and Loimaranta, 2000). Saliva acts a lubricant by neutralising and flushing out unwanted food particles from the tooth surface.

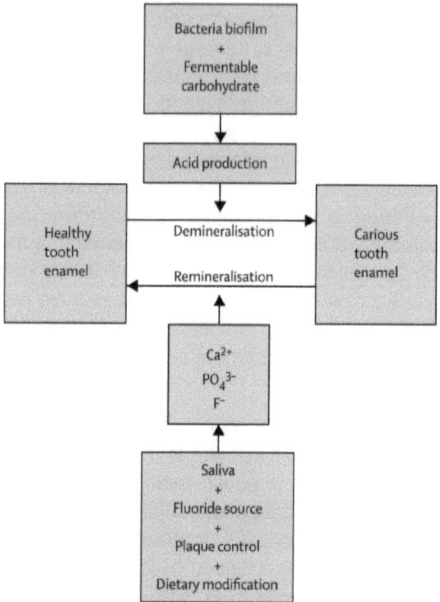

Figure 3:shows diagram of caries process as regular flux of demineralisation and remineralisation. Adapted from Kidd & Joyston-Bechal, 1997 (Kidd and Joyston-Bechal, 1997)

Toothpastes and mouthwashes are part of cosmetics that are beneficial in oral hygiene. Toothpastes and mouthwashes are cosmetic products used to clean, rinse, whiten, freshen and protect the teeth (Cury and Tenuta, 2014). Toothpaste is used together with toothbrush to prevent dental caries and promote good oral hygiene. In the absence of toothbrush in developing countries, a chewing stick or sponge is used ((Al-Otaibi et al., 2003). For example, in some parts of rural Ghana, the use of carved Neem tree or sponge as cleansing substances are still prevalent for cleaning the teeth. Researchers have stated that saliva also plays an important role in oral hygiene. Saliva is said to remove food debris through a buffering capacity and provide antimicrobial and antifungal effect which protects the enamel through the process of remineralisation (Lenander-Lumikari and Loimaranta, 2000).

The efficacy, quality and functionality of toothpaste have undergone diverse research and development stages in the past centuries (Cury and Tenuta, 2014). The functionality of toothpastes included the addition of ingredients that may chemically affect the tooth structure, reduce demineralisation, remove tartar, decrease hypersensitivity and provide antibacterial properties (Embery et al., 1992).

Most toothpastes usually contain natural and synthetic ingredients that may include glycerol, sodium lauryl sulphate, triclosan, sorbitol, fluoride, chlorhexidine etc (Stamm, 2007). Toothpastes and mouthwashes must have all the essential ingredients which help to maintain good oral hygiene by possessing the appropriate pH and abrasiveness (Cury and Tenuta, 2014).

1.3 Chemical agents

Fluoride is the most common ingredient used for the prevention of cavities on the teeth by providing protection to the enamel (Stamm, 2007). The use of toothpaste with fluoride was institutionalised in the developed countries by the 1960's to reduce demineralisation, promote remineralisation and good oral hygiene (Stamm, 2007, Twetman et al., 2003). Fluoride is the negative ion of the element fluorine, which is naturally found in human bones, teeth, plants, water, soil, and rocks. The benefits of fluoride are enormous. These may include:

I.   Controlling the growth of bacteria in the mouth

II.   Prevent mineral loss of the tooth enamel

III. Remineralise weak tooth enamel

The use of fluoride also impedes the metabolic process of bacteria by causing an instability in their cytoplasm (Chen et al., 2020).The main forms of fluoride present in toothpastes are sodium fluoride (0.245%, sodium monofluorophosphate (0.70%), amine fluoride (0.66%), stannous fluoride (0.454%) or a combination of any of them with a percentage concentration between 500-1500ppm (Twetman et al., 2003, Stamm, 2007). It is recommended that by way of practising good oral hygiene, the teeth should be brushed twice daily with a fluoridated toothpaste (Stamm, 2007, Tahmassebi et al., 2006). However, dentists, dental associations and public health experts recommend that "pea-sized" amount of toothpaste be administered to children under 6 years to reduce the rate of swallowing of the fluoride content in toothpaste (Davies et al., 2003). The tendency for children to swallow toothpaste is common and results in increased risk of enamel fluorosis, a change in appearance of the tooth enamel (Stamm, 2007).

With increased resistance of bacteria in the mouth, researchers progressed into finding and including Chlorhexidine as the "gold-standard" antiseptic for the removal of plaque (Fejerskov et al., 2015). Chlorhexidine, which is a cationic bis-biguanide has a strong affinity for tooth surfaces by disrupting the cell wall of the bacteria found in the mouth. Studies conducted in 1970 revealed that 01-0.2% of chlorhexidine could inhibit the antiplaque activity of mouth pathogens (Pemberton and Gibson, 2012). Xiugin Chen et al 2020, suggested that the ability of chlorhexidine to inhibit the development of plaque is by destroying the serosa permeability membrane of pathogens (Chen et al., 2020). The study highlighted high concentrations of chlorhexidine natures the cytoplasm of the pathogens and this mechanism results in inhibition of biofilm development. However, chlorhexidine has been reported to have several side effects such as staining of the teeth, discolouration of the tongue, mucosal soreness, desquamation, hypersensitivity, and bitter taste (Krishna et al., 2014). Scientists have stated that bacteria over time become resistant to chemicals such as chlorhexidine. There is reduced efficacy towards Gram-positive and Gram-negative bacteria (Horner et al., 2012). These side effects impose the need to find alternative sources that will be effective enamel protective agents in dentifrices.

1.4 Natural Products: Plant and marine extracts

As a result of increasing societal desire with the use of bioactive sources especially in healthcare, researchers have found the need to incorporate natural actives in dentifrice formulations. Aside from the use of fluoride and chlorhexidine as the means of protecting the enamel against dental caries and other cariogenic problems, natural sources such as Neem tree, seaweed, ginger, cloves, marine clay, kelp, ginseng have been researched to be effective towards the protection of the enamel by inhibiting the activity of oral bacteria (Jeon et al., 2011). A further example is, the novel production of activated charcoal whitening toothpaste to remove plaque from the tooth surface by Unilever. The use of natural ingredients in the cosmetic world has gained popularity since people believe it is safe, sustainable, cruelty-free and eco-friendly (Laroche et al., 2001, Dubey et al., 2004). There are unsubstantiated speculations that use of synthetic ingredients pose some side effects (Dubey et al., 2004). It has been widely viewed that the use of bioactive compounds in dentistry is less expensive, more potent, well tolerated, and safe. Therefore, the innovations of bioactive ingredients are essential. Natural ingredients originate from minerals, animals, leaves, soil, water, herbs etc. They provide nutritional benefits such as hydrocolloids, antimicrobial, preservatives, antioxidants, vitamins, proteins (Dubey et al., 2004).

With the increasing trend associated with the use of bioactive constituents, plants and marine algae have recently received attention due to their antimicrobial activity in dentistry. Aside from their uses as a source of nutrition in some parts of the world especially Asian countries, their ability of providing anti-allergy, anti-cancer, antimicrobial and anti-inflammation effects cannot be overemphasised (de Jesus Raposo et al., 2015). The world of marine algae, which is largely untapped has been found to consist of sesquiterpenes, phlorotannins, algal lectins, bromo-diterpenes and halogenated furanones that show antimicrobial effect against gram-positive and gram-negative bacteria (Swamy, 2011). These physiological effects of marine algae can be attributed to the presence of their polyphenolic components (Thomas and Kim, 2013)

Throughout history, natural products have exhibited effective and unconventional use for the control and prevention of many conditions (Jeon et al., 2011). In recent years, the interest in natural extracts in anti-caries research due to their bioactive molecules has seen a dramatic increase. Natural products exhibit pharmacodynamic properties by interacting with specific chemical receptors within the body and as such act as effective therapeutic agents (Seal et al., 2016). Therefore, exploiting alternative natural actives as preventive agents against dental caries will be appreciated by dentist, cosmetic formulators, and public health experts.

1.5 Problem Statement

Dental caries has become a public health problem. The prevalence of dental caries seems to be increasing worldwide and the most affected by this phenomenon are children, although adults are also greatly affected (Bagramian et al., 2009). Tooth decay is a public health threat because it leads to problems of malnutrition and other dental diseases (Bagramian et al., 2009). Discolouration of the teeth further tends to lower an individual's self-esteem (Grosofsky et al., 2003).

The process of acid influx, ingestion of extreme cold and warm substances can cause mineral loss (West and Joiner, 2014) and eventual wearing of the enamel.

Fluoride is needed to protect the enamel and prevent cavity formation (Davies et al., 2003) However, some individuals are extremely sensitive to the use of fluoride and others may consume it in high doses causing dental fluorosis (Osujp et al., 1988, Prabakar et al., 2019). Children under six years with ongoing teeth formation tend to have problems with dental fluorosis because of their poor swallowing mechanism (Davies et al., 2003).

Chlorhexidine has been used as a preventive agent against dental plaque and other oral health problems for many years now. However, its long-term use has been associated with bacterial resistance, bad taste in the mouth and teeth staining (Krishna et al., 2014). This means researchers must find safer, sustainable, eco-friendly effective alternative agents against dental caries. Natural extracts with bioactive sources have been researched to provide the effective alternative antimicrobial activity against oral pathogens (Freires et al., 2015).

Due to these undesirable side effects of Chlorhexidine and the constant scrutiny with the use of fluoride in dentifrices, this review will through literature investigate innovative natural sources of marine and plant bioactive components against dental caries as alternative anticaries agents.

1.6 Aim

This review will explore biological active sources of marine and plant extracts that protect the enamel through their antimicrobial activity against cariogenic bacteria.

1.6.1 Objectives
1. To investigate the biological activity of natural extracts
2. To examine the mechanism of inhibition of plaque by pathogens
3. To provide natural alternative sources against biofilm formation as compared to fluoride and chlorhexidine.

1.6.2 Review Questions
I.   Will bioactive sources of plant and marine extracts protect the enamel by being effective against cariogenic pathogens?
II. Will inhibition of oral pathogens result in remineralisation of the tooth enamel?

1.7 Limitations of This Study

This review will provide the necessary literature and knowledge of anti-caries natural extracts even though information on the topic may be limited.

Due to biodiversity, uncertain seasonal and environmental conditions, the continuity, and reproducibility of some natural actives for cosmetic formulation may be difficult.

1.8 Significance of Study:

According to Robert V. Faller et al, "Tooth health can be measured not only by prevention against subsurface damage (caries), but also by assessing the ability of products to strengthen and protect enamel against acid-induced tooth softening that can lead to irreversible erosive tooth damage" (Faller et al., 2011). This quote suggests that there should be consistent research to find new natural actives for enamel protection. This review seeks to find biological active extracts from natural products which may have not been explored adequately. For example, the British Dental Journal in August of 2012 published an article titled "Is seaweed superior to toothpaste" (Pacey, 2012). In the article, a team of dentists and scientists from Newcastle University were in the process of developing a cleaning product which could a better replacement for plaque removal and cavity protection as compared to conventional toothpaste. According to Dubey et al, 2004, plant extracts for therapeutic and commercial purposes have not been exploited (Dubey et al., 2004).

This review is therefore intended to provide a consolidated source of evidence to inform readers and consumers of the benefits of bioactive extracts in the prevention of dental caries and the need to protect the enamel.

This review will contribute to the knowledge in the cosmetic industry on enamel protection since it will aim at finding biological active components in the natural ingredients that could be effective towards the control of dental caries or plaque.

The number of dentifrices with natural actives formulation on the market is very low and hence this review seeks to explore new marine and plant bioactive sources as variety of dentifrices formulation for consumers.

This review can be used by manufacturers in cosmetic industry for the research and development of toothpastes and mouthwashes formulations.

This review also intends to inform consumers of the benefits of maintaining regular good oral hygiene

1.9 Scope of Study

This review will be involved in the use of literature to explore plant and marine extracts only and their effectiveness towards the prevention of dental caries, plaque, tartar, and gingivitis.

The use of animals and nanoparticles is excluded from this review. This review excludes the literature of the dentine and pulp as conditions affecting them may not be considered as cosmetic conditions.

CHAPTER TWO: RESEARCH METHODOLOGY

A systematic literature review was conducted on existing literature relating to natural actives and its effect on dental carries.

Articles that were relevant to this review were retrieved from Google scholar and Science Direct databases. The scope of this review included old publications dated as far back as 1989 to enable outline the process of research made by scientists and researchers on the control and prevention of dental caries. With 19000 articles identified, 40 articles fulfilled the selection criteria. The articles selected mentioned natural products/actives with emphasis on dental caries or anti-caries effect.

To select relevant articles, a selection criterion was established. A combination of keywords of Boolean operators such as "AND", "ON" and "OR" were used to search text terms. For example, natural actives and dental caries. The keyword "effect" was added to the search term to capture all relevant articles. For example, effect of natural actives on dental caries.

The initial database search identified 19000 results. The second stage involved a brief assessment of the title and abstract of the articles produced and out of that, 18950 were excluded. In the next stage, a search method was used to verify how natural extracts and dental caries were mentioned in the article. The number of times this was mentioned in the article was a critical decider for inclusion and exclusion. This is because some articles only mentioned natural actives or dental caries once in the article. Lastly, 40 papers were selected and used for this review based on the information on the aims and objectives of the study.

The processes involved in the content selection was used to assess the knowledge of literature in the subject area. The first step involved understanding the effect natural products had on caries prevention. The second step involved assessing the mechanisms involved in dental caries formation and the last step involved merging the ideas to create a cohesive and logical theme for the review.

Dr Eric Duodu, a Dentist at the Glamordent Lighthouse Dental Practice, Withernsea near Hull was also consulted to enquire about the different conditions that may affect the enamel and on the use of natural products in dentistry.

Snowballing, which applies to the process where references of the located article is also beneficial towards the aims and objectives for the review. This process helped to find useful sources of information relating to the topic of *"oral care", "dental caries", "oral hygiene", "plant extracts in oral care", marine extracts in oral care", "seaweed in oral care", marine extracts in dental caries", "enamel demineralisation", "effect of fluoride in toothpaste", "marine extracts and dental caries"* etc.

For the best of results in literature, the focus was on articles containing laid out experimental and analytical procedures indicating the outcome of the effectiveness of natural actives on cariogenic bacteria and further to provide alternative preventive agents compared to fluoride and chlorhexidine.

Consideration for the credibility, validity and reliability of the sources were also noted in the process. A list of factors that were considered during the search were:

i.   Is the information organised and clear enough?

ii.   Is the information accurate?

iii.   Has the information been cited on numerous occasions for research?

iv.   Has the information been based on previous work?

With all these questions properly answered, the sources of information were chosen. Sources of information which were found to be decades old were used to establish fundamental concepts in current research.

CHAPTER THREE: RESULTS AND FINDINGS

As stated in the earlier section, dental carries can be detrimental to human health and therefore preventive agents should be used to prevent and control its occurrence. Natural products have used for treatment of different ailments over the years (Jafari et al., 2018). In 2015, dental caries was ranked the third most prevalent disease with a cost of €90 billion (Chen et al., 2020).

The control and prevention of caries is critical in public health management to enable individuals have a healthy tooth structure (Chen et al., 2020). Through research, natural products have been studied and proven to exhibit antimicrobial activity against dental caries (Lee et al., 2019). In this section, natural products that exert antimicrobial activity through their bioactive sources will be explored.

3.1 Causes and effect of dental caries

Lifestyle habits such as diet has been accounted to play a significant role in the development of dental caries. (Fejerskov et al., 2015). Bacterial fermentation of dietary carbohydrates deposit acid onto the enamel destroying its hard tissues. However, Barima Islam et al suggests that the first point of dental caries is negligence of oral hygiene (Islam et al., 2008).

Environmental factors such as temperature, pH conditions, salinity and oxygen cause a drop in pH affecting the salivation in the mouth and contribute to the formation of biofilms/plaque formation on the enamel (Takahashi and Nyvad, 2010). Marsh & Nyvad 2008 stated that demineralisation of the enamel can be attributed to low pH and acid production resulting from carbohydrate metabolism (Marsh, 2005)., however they are different opinions regarding the causes of dental caries such as physiological traits of plaque contributing to the process of demineralisation.

According to research over the years, *S. mutans* are the main causative bacteria of dental caries. They play four major roles in the process of dental caries: firstly; its separation from lesions of cavitated caries, secondly; the process of excessive sugar intake leading to plaque formation, thirdly; the deposit of acid on the tooth surface and lastly; the adhesion of bacteria to the enamel by water-insoluble glucans (Takahashi and Nyvad, 2010). The processes stated indicate the role of *S. mutans* as the main causative agent in dental caries (Tanzer et al).

Sajith Vellappally et al suggested that there is relationship between smoking and dental caries (Vellappally et al., 2007). It was also stated that smokers tend to ignore regular brushing and flossing of the teeth (Vellappally et al., 2007). Some other researchers also supported this assertion and have stated that a drop in salivary pH of smokers coupled with increased number of *S. mutans and Lactobacilli* enhances a smoker's vulnerability to dental caries (Johnson and Bain, 2000). However, other researchers were against this opinion and believed that the concentration of thiocyanate in tobacco increases salivary flow and therefore tobacco smoking decreased a smoker's chances of dental caries effect (Johnson and Bain, 2000). Due to different opinions, it is difficult to establish a stronger aetiological relationship between smoking and dental caries.

Khushbu Yadav et al highlighted in 2017 that dry mouth and eating disorders also contributes to dental caries occurrence. When there is dehydration of saliva in the mouth which may be due to the intake of certain medications, acid is produced from bacteria resulting in biofilm formation. Eating disorders also contribute to dental caries and erosion by releasing stomach acids which breaks down the enamel (Yadav and Prakash, 2017).

3.2 Prevention and Control

Chlorhexidine, fluoride, and other ingredients in toothpaste such as triclosan, sodium lauryl sulphate and hydrated silica have been used ingredients in toothpaste to control cavities, provide fresh breath and aid in whitening the teeth. However, as consumers become more interested in integrating natural actives in toothpastes, manufacturers have found the need to incorporate these ingredients in their toothpaste formulations. However, some of these new and innovative ways to enhance good oral health has been around since periods of ancient Greek (Greenwall et al., 2019). One of these traditions is the use of charcoal to clean the teeth (Greenwall et al., 2019). Charcoal is a fine grain powder made from wood and other natural substances that help to remove tartar from the enamel (Greenwall et al., 2019) by means of absorption and has been touted as one of the surest ways of cleaning the enamel. With the word 'natural' becoming pronounced in recent times and the need to control the prevalence of dental caries, researchers have resorted greatly to the marine world for its abundance of unique bioactive components and benefits (Thomas and Kim, 2013). Extracts from plants are also undergoing numerous research for the prevention of dental caries (Philip et al., 2019).

3.3 Plant extracts in caries prevention

JJ Hannah et al in 1989 conducted an experimental study, where 24 subjects were subjected to a six-month period of evaluation to assess the efficacy of sanguinaria against the control of plaque and gingivitis. The process was assessed using the Silness and Loe plaque index and Loe and Silness gingival index throughout the 6 months period. The results indicated that there was a reduction of plaque and gingival formation by 51% and 60% respectively when subjects used the sanguinaria for brushing within the stipulated period. A repeated analytical process indicated the significant reduction of plaque and gingivitis within a 6-month period. With a combined use of sanguinaria containing toothpaste and mouth rinse, the results showed a significant reduction of biofilms and gingivitis (Hannah et al., 1989).

Camellia sinensis (Theaceae) is made up of three main teas which *oolong tea, black tea,* and *green tea. In vivo* analysis performed by Asmat Rasheed et al revealed that the extracts of *Camellia sinensis* was effective at inhibiting cariogenic bacteria, *S. mutans, Streptococcus salivarius* and *E. coli* as compared to *amoxicillin, cephradine* and *eugenol* (Rasheed and Haider, 1998).

Development of therapeutic agents with antimicrobial properties is one sure method of reducing the incidence of dental caries. This was proven by Nostro et al 2004 when the team conducted an *in-vitro* study to assess the concentrations of *Helichrysum italicum* extract that will be effective against cariogenic pathogens. *H. italicum* is a plant commonly found in the Mediterranean region with researched biological properties such as antiallergic, anti-inflammatory and antimicrobial properties. The study involved three oral pathogens *S. mutans, S. salivarius* and *S. sanguis*. The results revealed that the ethanolic extracts of the plant were effective against all the three tested oral pathogens. However, the highest efficacy was against *S. mutans* (Nostro et al., 2004).

M. Raveendra Pai et al conducted a 6-week clinical study in 2004 to examine the antimicrobial activity of Neem extract (*Azadirachta indica*) against *S. mutans* and *Lactobacilli spp.* using a chlorhexidine gluconate 0.2% mouthwash as the positive control. After the semi-quantitative four quadrant streaking method, the results indicated that the tannin components in *Azadirachta indica* were effective against the two strains of cariogenic bacteria and therefore suggested that Neem extract is a possible source to consider as an anti-caries agent (Pai et al., 2004).

To test the polyphenolic components of Hop bract extract against dental caries, Shinada et al, 2007 conducted a double-blind crossover clinical study to ascertain the effect of the extract in humans. Twenty-nine male volunteers used the prepared 0.1% Hop bract polyphenol mouth rinse against a placebo. The results conclusively indicated a positive inhibition of glucosyltransferases, which is responsible for the growth of *S. mutans*. Hop bract extract can therefore be considered as a promising agent for the control of dental caries (Shinada et al., 2007).

To effectively destroy the acidogenicity pathways of *S. mutans*, its sugar transport enzymatic activity, proton motive force and glycolytic mechanism should be targeted. An experiment to investigate this cause was explored by Gregoire et al in 2007. In this *in vitro* study, a semi-preparative high-performance liquid chromatography method was used to isolate the flavonols, phenols and proanthocyanidins from Cranberry fruit (*Vaccinium macrocarpon*) extract. The report indicated that the Cranberry extract consisted of quercetin-3-arabinofuranoside, mycertin and procyanidin A2 bioactive components, which was responsible for the inhibition of glucosyltransferases by 15-30% and the disruption of the acidogenicity of the *S. mutans*. However, Gregoire et al 2007 stated that the bioactive components effect on *S. mutans* was because of the combination of activity from all the three bioactive compounds. Cranberry extract was therefore reported to inhibit the glycolytic enzymatic activity of *S. mutans* and should be considered for its cariostatic property (Gregoire et al., 2007).

Poureslami et al, 2008 adopted a three-way experimental process to evaluate the antibacterial effect of miswak extracts on dental plaque. Firstly, an analysis to assess the concentration of the miswak extracts that will exert its antibacterial properties. Secondly, an experiment to determine the antibacterial effects of the miswak extract and a placebo toothpaste from an Iranian company was conducted. Twelve subjects were involved in the process. The results of the *in vitro* test showed a significance effectiveness of the miswak extract against the placebo toothpaste by 13.63%. The last step of experiment involved the miswak extracts, and a Swiss toothpaste known as Quail miswak to ascertain the antibacterial effects on *three (3) causative bacteria* of plaque namely *S. sanguis, S. sobrinus, S. salivarius* and *Actinomyces viscous*. Then the miswak extracts combined with the Quail miswak was assessed against penicillin. The results from the miswak extracts indicated a significant efficacy towards plaque removal as compared to the penicillin. Poureslami et al's study showed a significant difference when the herbal extracts were employed as compared to specimen without the extracts. The antibacterial effect of the miswak extract against dental plaque was enormous and maybe employed in dentifrices (Poureslami et al., 2008).

To assess the effectiveness of *Mentha spicata* and *eucalyptus camaldulensis* as essential oils against a placebo dentifrice formulated with chlorhexidine on plaque was carried out by I. Rasooli et al in 2009. Using *in vitro* and *in vivo* methods, the antimicrobial effects of the oils on plaque were analysed. The method of the analysis used was gas chromatography and gas chromatography mass spectrometry involving 15 compounds of the *Mentha spicata* and 21 compounds of the *e. camaldulensis*. Interpretation of the results proved that the essential oils had higher efficacy of antimicrobial activities for the removal of plaque as compared to that of chlorhexidine. However, the *in vivo* study was conducted in Iran and therefore could not be a generalisation of the world's population. Another problem involved the assessment of the subjects undergoing the *in vivo* study. The review process was conducted only once a week which could have allowed for any of them to use a different toothpaste. Nonetheless, the process to indicate the effectiveness of the essential oils against plaque formation was achieved (Rasooli et al., 2009).

F. C Sampaio et al, 2009 investigated the antimicrobial activity of *Caesalpinia ferrea* martius fruits against oral pathogen. In the study, 'H NMR was used to extract methanol for to assess the polyphenolic components of the fruits. Using chlorhexidine as the positive control, the microdilution method of the planktonic cells was used to test the causative agents of dental plaque namely, *S. mutans, S. salivarius, Candida albicans, Streptococcus oralis* and *Lactobacillus casei.* The result of the *in vitro* assay indicated that polyphenols extracted from the *Caesalpinia ferrea* fruits inhibited the growth of oral pathogens (Sampaio et al., 2009).

Using both the agar diffusion and both methods, F. Sedighinia et al, 2012 conducted an *in vitro* study on glycyrrhiza glabra to assess its antimicrobial activity on oral bacteria. The microorganisms used in the analysis were *Escherichia coli, Enterococcus faecalis,* S. mutans, Actinomyces viscosus, *Staphylococcus aureus* and S. sanguis. The results indicated that the ethanolic extract of the glycyrrhiza glabra inhibited the growth of the microorganisms (Sedighinia and Afshar, 2012).

Skaba et al, 2013 also proved that propolis extract supports the removal of dental plaque from tooth enamel during their cohort study to evaluate the effect of Brazilian extract of propolis (EEP) on the oral cavity. The study involved 32 patients (17 females and 15 males). The group was divided into two categories according to the state of their dental caries. 50mg/L of the EEP was used as the concentration to assess the antimicrobial activity against the removal of dental plaque. assessment of the results was based on three indexes which were approximal plaque index (API), oral hygiene index (OHI) and sulcus bleeding index (SBI). At the end of the study, they observed that the concentration of the EEP extracted was effective towards the removal of dental plaque to protect the enamel. The study however failed to state the ages of the subjects involved which may have had an influencing factor on the process (Skaba et al., 2013).

13

M. Prasanth et al, developed a study to determine the antibacterial activity of six herbal toothpastes on Gram-positive bacteria *S. mutans*, *Lactobacilli acidophilus* and fungus *Candida albicans* using *in vitro* methods. The results which were determined by the agar well diffusion method indicated that all the six herbal toothpastes were effective against cariogenic pathogens. The combination of dried ginger, black pepper, long pepper, Herra, liquorice, Kapoor and cloves showed the highest efficacy. However, the study did not state the inclusion of a placebo toothpaste for comparison (Prasanth and Ratha, 2014).

Consequently, the use of propolis extract in the dental field has been growing and Bhat et al, 2015 proved this assertion in their study which aimed at determining the antimicrobial efficacy of propolis extract for its anti-plaque properties. The crossover clinical study involved 30 dental students who were tested on a toothpaste containing propolis extract against a Colgate toothpaste and a miswak toothpaste for a period of two weeks. The students used a washout product to cleanse their teeth to remove any debris of food particles or contaminants that may alter the results of the study. They were then made to brush their teeth with the formulated propolis extract toothpaste. After 24 hours, the results showed that propolis formulated dentifrice was the best in the removal of the plaque as compared to the miswak and Colgate toothpaste (Bhat et al., 2015).

In a randomised clinical trial study, Beheshti-Rouy et al, 2015 explored the effect of sage extracts (*Salvia officinalis*) in a mouthwash against *S. mutans*. Seventy students, both males and females were selected from a school and divided into two groups equally. The first group used the preparation of mouthwash made from the sage extracts whiles the second group used a placebo mouthwash without any anti-cariogenic ingredients. After twenty-one days of assessing the outcome of the trial, the statistical data analysis was conducted using the t-student tests with $p<0.05$ to evaluate the significance levels. The results positively indicated that sage extracts contained monoterpenoids which were responsible for their antimicrobial effect in the disruption of the dental plaque. It was confirmed that sage extracts were efficacious in the inhibition of *S. mutans* and therefore should be considered as a potential source of anti-caries agent in oral healthcare. However, this study was carried out in Iran and therefore may not be a representation of all individuals in the world (Beheshti-Rouy et al., 2015).

In 2016, *Mikania glomerata*, a plant mainly found in Brazil was evaluated against dental caries by Moreira et al, 2016. The diterpenoid properties of the plant were stated to be responsible for its antimicrobial, antiallergy, bronchodilating and anti-inflammatory properties. To evaluate its antimicrobial properties against cariogenic

bacteria, the HPLC-DAD method was used to assess it kaurenoic acid (KA). In the *in vitro* study chlorhexidine digluconate was used as the positive control. The results of the KA showed a higher inhibition against the microorganisms proving that the KA extract of the plant can be considered as a natural anti-caries ingredient. However, the chlorhexidine digluconate also indicated higher efficacy against the oral pathogens (Moreira et al., 2016).

The extracts from jujube leaves have been investigated for its antimicrobial effect for the prevention of dental caries by Damiano et al in 2017. A 2,2-diphenyl-1-picrylhydrazyl (DPPH) guided purification study identified lupane triterpenoid alphitolic acid as the antimicrobial agent in jujube leaves which is responsible for its antibiofilm activity. The result also indicated that the concentration of polyphenol present in the extract could coordinate with the alphitolic acid through pharmacokinetic process to exert its antiplaque effect and therefore did not alter the biosynthetic pathways of the oral the cavity. At the end, the study proved that Ziziphus jujube leaves had antimicrobial activity against cariogenic bacteria and therefore should be considered as a possible anticaries agent (Damiano et al., 2017).

An *in vitro* study to determine the polyphenolic activity of Pomegranate peel and juice as an anti-caries agent was conducted by G. F Ferrazzano et al in 2017. Under the reverse phase HPLC (RP) and mass spectrometry the minimum inhibitory concentration (MIC) and minimum bacterial concentration (MBC) were evaluated. These standards were assessed against two strains of cariogenic bacteria-*S. mutans* ATCC 25175 and *Rotinia dentocariosa* clinical isolate. The results indicated that the polyphenolic and hydroalcoholic components of the juice and peel demonstrated greater efficacy in the inhibition of caries (Ferrazzano et al., 2017).

Thai traditional herbs against oral pathogens were tested for their antibacterial and antibiofilm activity by R. Teanpaisan et al in 2017. Twelve ethanol extracts were obtained from all the different plant extracts and were evaluated using the agar well diffusion, broth microdilution and time-kill methods. Using the 3-(4,5-dimethyl-2-thiazolyl)-2,5-diphenyl-2H-tetrazolium-bromide (MTT) assay, the antibiofilm activity was assessed. Among all the plant extracts, *Piper Betle* showed the highest antimicrobial property towards the causative bacteria. *Piper Betle* contained 4-chromanol, which was responsible for the antibacterial and antibiofilm activity against oral bacteria (Teanpaisan et al., 2017).

3.4 Marine extracts in oral care

The use of marine extracts for oral hygiene has also been growing and investigated over the past decades. For example, seaweeds have used for health and nutritional benefits especially in Asian countries. Seaweeds which are sometimes called Kelp comprise of brown, green, and red algae (Kandale et al., 2011)

Dried mushroom extract of *Lentinus edodes* (Shiitake) were examined to determine its antibacterial activity against oral pathogens by M. Hirasawa et al in 1999. The antibacterial activity was anaerobically determined using the gas-substitution method. The results showed that when the extracts were subjected to the pathogens, there was significant reduction of the water-insoluble glucans. Therefore, the study revealed the effectiveness of *Lentinus edodes* extracts as positive anti-caries agent (Hirasawa et al., 1999).

Crustacean shells contain chitosan (1-4, 2-amino-2-deoxy-β-Ð-glucan) which has been researched for its antimicrobial properties. For its use an anti-caries agent, H J Busscher et al investigated the antimicrobial effects of chitosan in crustaceans against dental plaque. Chitosan being polycationic tends to bind well to salivary pellicles and therefore reduce the effectiveness of *Streptococcus sanguinis* on the enamel. The results indicated that chitosan was a viable natural source for the prevention of pathogens such as *S. sanguinis* (Busscher et al., 2008).

L. Sujatha et al, 2012 demonstrated that green seaweeds consisted of antibacterial activity against oral bacteria. Four species of the green seaweeds namely, *Chaetomorphia antenina, Cladophora fascularis, Spongomorpha indica* and *Ulva fasciata* were tested on three oral bacteria-*S. mutans, Streptococcus mitis* and *Actinomyces viscosus*. Using the agar diffusion method, the results confirmed that the methanolic extracts of the seaweeds inhibited the oral pathogens and the antibacterial properties were highly effective for preventing dental caries (Sujatha et al., 2012).

In the study of Yeon-Hee Kim et al, the antimicrobial activity of ethanol extracts of *Laminaria japonica* (a type of seaweed) for the removal of dental plaque was assessed. The results revealed that ethanol extract concentrations of laminaria japonica was effective on *S. mutans* and *Porphyromonas gingivalis* (Kim et al., 2013).

Jun et al investigated the antimicrobial and antibiofilm activities of sulphated polysaccharides from eight marine algae against oral pathogens. The acid extraction method was used to evaluate the polysaccharides. *Fucus vesoculosus* with the fucoidan concentration above 250µg/mL exhibited the highest suppression of the biofilms when tested against the oral bacteria, *S. mutans* and *S. sobrinus* (Jun et al., 2018).

S. Jafari et al, 2018 performed an *in vitro* analysis to determine the antibacterial and antibiofilm activity of *Chlorella vulgaris* and *Dunaliella salina* against *S. mutans* using the disc diffusion, well diffusion, MIC, and MBC methods. The results confirmed that the two microalgae consist of flavonoids, tannins and terpenes that were responsible for the anti-caries activity. It was concluded that *Chlorella vulgaris* and *Dunaliella salina* were efficacious against *S. mutans (Jafari et al., 2018).*

Kelp, which is another type of seaweed belonging to the family of brown algae has gained popularity in the oral healthcare field with its antimicrobial property showing significant efficacy against biofilms (Oka et al., 2020). Fucoidans, a type of kelp was assessed and determined to have antimicrobial activity against *S. mutans*, in an *in vitro* study conducted by S. Oka et al in 2020.

Several published studies have explored the use of natural extracts in dentistry and have indicated their effectiveness against cariogenic bacteria. However, the process of identification, isolation, purification, and characterisation has proven to be complex (Jeon et al., 2011). With the use of bioactive sources to prevent dental caries been less costly as compared to conventional use of fluoride or chlorhexidine, there is the need for extensive research to identify new bioactive sources to enable dentists, consumers, health care practitioners and policy makers find solutions during decision making. A summary of the selected key natural products, their bioactive compounds, and mechanisms of anticaries is presented in table 1 below.

Table 1:Table of natural products showing their biological activity as alternative anticaries agents

References	Source of natural product	Bioactive component	Outcome/Biological activity
JJ Hannah et al 1989	Sanguinaria extract	Sanguinarine	-antimicrobial activity against *S. mutans*
Asmat Rasheed et al 1998	Camellia sinensis	Catechin, epigallocatechin gallate, saponins	Inhibition of *S. mutans* and *S. salivarius* -inhibitory effect on glucosyltransferase activity and acidogenicity
A. Nostro et al 2003	*Helichrysum italicum* extract (Curry plant)	Polyphenols	-antimicrobial activity against *S. mutans*
M. Raveendra Pai et al 2004	*Azadirachta indica* (Neem extract)	Tannins	-antibacterial activity against water-insoluble glucans
Poureslami et al 2007	miswak extracts	Unknown	-antimicrobial activity against S. mutans
Shinada et al 2007	Hop bract	Polyphenols	-Inhibition of glucosyltransferases
Gregoire et al 2007	Cranberry fruit	Flavonols, phenols and proanthocyanidins	-inhibition of glucosyltransferases -disruption of acidogenicity pathway of *S. mutans*
I. Rasooli et al 2009	Mentha spicata and eucalyptus camaldulensis (Essential oils)	Terpinene	-Inhibition of plaque
Fabio C. Sampaio et al 2009	Caesalpinia ferrea martius fruit	Polyphenols	-inhibition of activity of cariogenic bacteria including *S. mutans*
Fereshteh Sedighinia et al 2012	Glycyrrhiza glabra	Polyphenols	-antibacterial activity against oral bacteria

Manupati Prasanth et al 2014	Six herbal extract- dried ginger, black pepper, long pepper, herra, liquorice, karpoor and cloves	Unknown	-inhibition of cariogenic bacteria
Maryam Beheshti-Rouy et al 2015	Sage extract	Monoterpenoid	-disruption of dental plaque
Monique Rodrigues et al 2016	Mikania glomerata	Kaurenoic acid	-antimicrobial activity against oral pathogens
Silvia Damiano et al 2017	Jujube leaves	Polyphenols	-antimicrobial activity against cariogenic bacteria
Gianmaria Fabrizio et al 2017	Pomegranate juice and peel	Polyphenols	-inhibition of activity of cariogenic bacteria including *S. mutans*
Rawee Teanpaisan et al 2017	Piper Betle	4-chromatol	-antimicrobial and antibiofilm activity against oral bacteria
Marine Extracts			
Masatomo Hirasawa et al 1999	Lentinus edodes (Shiitake)	Lenthionine	-inhibition of water-insoluble glucans
Henk J. Busscher et al 2008	Crustacean shells	Chitoologosaccharide	-antimicrobial and antibiofilm activity against planktonic oral pathogens, *S. sanguis*
L. Sujatha et al 2012	Four species of green seaweeds: *Chaetomorphia antenina*, *Cladophora fascularis*, *Spongomorpha indica* and *Ulva fasciata*	Methanolic extracts	-antibacterial properties against cariogenic bacteria

Yeon-Hee Kim et al 2013	Laminaria japonica	Sulphated polysaccharide	-inhibition of dental plaque
Joon-Young Jun et al 2018	Fucus vesiculosus (Fucoidans)	Fucoidans	-inhibition of oral bacteria biofilm
Shima Jafari et al 2018	Chlorella vulgaris and Dunaliella salina	Flavonoids, Tannins, and terpenes	-antibacterial activity against *S. mutans*
Shunya Oka et al 2019	Kelp	Fucoidans	-antimicrobial activity against *S. mutans*

CHAPTER FOUR: DISCUSSION

4.1 Interpretation of findings

Dental caries is the most prevailing dental condition worldwide (Prabakar et al). Caries formation has been associated with the existence of biofilms. Extracellular polymeric substances (EPS) are natural polymers that create a viable environment for biofilms to exist (Chen et al., 2020). EPS promote the virulence of pathogens by creating habitats for acid production. A combination of microorganisms comprises of the formation of biofilms even though *S. mutans* are the main causative agents (Jeon et al., 2011). These microorganisms secrete fermented carbohydrates through the enzymatic activity of glucosyltransferase to synthesize EPS. Glucosyltransferases are enzymes that utilize fermented sugar to form soluble and insoluble glucans on the tooth surface (Koo et al., 2002). The glucans aid in the adherence and accumulation of S. mutans to the enamel. As *S. mutans* thrive longer on the enamel, there is significant development from plaque formation to caries formation (Koo et al., 2002, Jeon et al., 2011). The structure of EPS provides stability and protection for biofilms to survive and promote the virulence of pathogens by creating binding sites for acid production (Chen et al., 2020). The activity of EPS also creates a low-pH environment for pathogens to exist which results in demineralisation of the enamel (Jeon et al., 2011). These conditions are critical for the development of biofilms and therefore inhibition of the activity of GTF on the enamel is one of the strategies to prevent and control dental caries (Jeon et al., 2011).

From the literature gathered, there seems to be natural products that possess anticaries properties. Natural products have been in use for many years to control, prevent and treat most ailments including oral conditions (Ajagannanavar et al., 2014). Naturally occurring bioactive compound have always been explored for the development of drugs and cosmetics due to its high chemical and biochemical constituents present in their structures (Philip et al., 2019). These chemical structures may be categorised as to whether they contain nitrogen or not and secondly, whether they contain rings with sugar moieties or not (Chinou, 2008). Natural products contain secondary metabolites that are obtained from organisms and this help to fight pathogens and other undesirable attacks (Singer et al., 2003). It has been estimated that plants produce 500,000 secondary metabolites (Singer et al., 2003). Based on the chemical structures from the secondary metabolites of these natural products, their phytochemical sources have been classified into three (Jeon et al., 2011):

I.   Alkaloids: are nitrogen-containing compounds. Example sanguinarine

II.   Polyphenols: they are mostly found in the plant kingdom and are made from simple sugars containing benzene rings, hydrogen, and oxygen (e.g., flavonoids of propolis)

III. Terpenoids: they are mostly comprised of hydrogen and carbon from mevalonic acid. Mostly essential oils used in dentifrices (e.g., Eugenol and thymol).

These bioactive components of natural products have been associated with antioxidants, anticancer and antimicrobial properties (Newmann et al). The antimicrobial properties of natural products demonstrate their effect on pathogens through three major mechanisms (Jeon et al., 2011). Firstly, the inhibition of pathogenic growth through antimicrobial properties, secondly, the inhibition of glucosyltransferase synthesis, and lastly, the disruption of biofilm adherence to the tooth. Aside from these three ways of disruption mechanisms, natural products should provide rich sources of non-fermentable sugars to balance the relationship between remineralisation and demineralisation process (Philip et al., 2019)

Compared to chlorhexidine, naturally occurring biological active compounds exhibit high affinity of inhibitory effects against *S. mutans* (Rasooli et al., 2009). For example, the minimum inhibitory concentrations (MIC) of essential oils against cariogenic bacteria. The chemical structures of essential oils consist of low molecular weight terpenes, terpenoids, aliphatic and aromatic compounds that are responsible for their antimicrobial properties (Dorman and Deans, 2000). The ability of essential oils to breakdown the lipids of bacterial cell wall of pathogens is due to their hydrophilic nature. They destroy the pathogenic membrane and cause leakage to the cell proteins leading to cell death (Jeon et al., 2011). For example, the inhibition of cariogenic pathogens by thymol and eugenol.

The research of polyphenols indicates a potential inhibitory effect on biofilms due to their antimicrobial properties. For example, *Helichrysum italicum* (curry plant), commonly found in the Mediterranean region contain rich sources of polyphenols identified to inhibit water-insoluble glucans. Cranberry extracts, propolis, tea and Neem (Azadirachta indica) collectively consists of different types of polyphenols such as flavonoids, proanthocyanidins, apigenin and gallotannins that contribute to caries prevention (Philip et al., 2019). The components of the polyphenols inhibit the activity of GTF by reducing the acid synthesis of insoluble glucans. This process should be successfully achieved without disturbing the viability of the oral region (Philip et al., 2019).

Marine extracts, *Lentinus edodes* (Shiitake) is mostly located in Asia and usually consumed raw or cooked have been documented to possess rich sources of Lenthionine (Hirasawa et al., 1999). When consumed regularly, this could decrease the incidence of caries by the release of its antimicrobial properties. The main components of Lenthionine and the disulphide derivatives in Shiitake are responsible for its inhibitory effect. These compounds stop the supply of oxygen to *S. mutans* resulting in an unstable and unfunctional cell membrane (Hirasawa et al., 1999)

Pomegranate juice and peel has been identified to possess pharmacological properties such as the ability to scavenge free radicals due its rich polyphenolic content (ellagitannins and anthocyanins). In traditional medicine, Pomegranate has been used to treat diarrhoea, respiratory pathogens, and dysentery (Ferrazzano et al., 2017). It's peel and juice extracts have shown effective antimicrobial properties against the inhibition of oral pathogens (Pagliarulo et al., 2016). Priya Subramaniam et al also supported this assertion through an in vitro study of the antibacterial activity of Pomegranate extract against cariogenic bacteria (Subramaniam et al., 2012).

Chlorella vulgaris and *Dunaliella salina* are microalgae with rich supply of proteins, vitamins and minerals (Zheng et al., 2012). *D. salina* are flagellate microalgae usually found in sea salt and salty lake and are halophile green unicellular in nature (Hosseini Tafreshi and Shariati, 2009). Studies have shown that they exhibit antioxidant activity due to its richness in carotenoids. *Chlorella vulgaris* species extracts have been researched to consist of terpenoids, alkaloids, cyclic peptides and tannins which are responsible for their antibacterial activities against oral pathogens (Zheng et al., 2012). A report by Marjorie Murphy Cowan stated that the reaction between oxidised compounds and sulfhydryl groups are the chief active components of the phenolic antibacterial activity (Cowan, 1999). Alkaloids and terpenes have been reported as strong active agents against pathogens. Flavonoids, tannins, phenolic compounds, terpenoids and saponins have been researched by Uma et al as the most active antibacterial agents against *Streptococcus aureus* (Desbois and Smith, 2010). The actual phytochemical constituent that exhibits these prohibitive effects on *S. mutans* are unknown, however, it is believed that the hydrophilic compounds of the terpenoids penetrate the bacterial cell wall, cause a disruption in electron transfer, and prohibits the supply of oxygen resulting in a collapse of bacterial cells (Jafari et al., 2018).

Sanguinaria is a plant extract obtained from the rhizomes of the bloodroot plant *Sanguinaria canadensis.* Th extract is made up of alkaloid compounds of benzophenanthridine with a positive electron charge which is responsible for its plaque inhibition and reduction in gingival inflammation (Bonesvoll and Gjermo, 1978).

Factors such as adhesion, acidogenicity and aciduricity generally affect the activity of certain phytochemical compounds (Philip et al., 2019). The phenolic content of Cranberry juice, however, has been suggested to be able to decrease the acidogenicity produced by cariogenic bacteria, *S. mutans* (Duarte et al., 2006). The use of natural actives over the years have shown to be effective to disrupt the sucrose-dependent and sucrose-independent pathogenic adhesion to the tooth enamel (Islam et al., 2008, Badet and Quero, 2011). Natural actives have shown to reduce the average mass of plaque formation without disturbing the presence of good mouth bacteria (Busscher et al., 2008). For example, chitosans which is obtained from shells of crustaceans is a marine source that have been researched to inhibit the adhesion of oral pathogens on the tooth enamel. Natural extracts also have shown to promote remineralisation of the enamel by inhibiting the formation of dental plaque (Beheshti-Rouy et al., 2015). For example, Sage extracts (*Salvia officinalis*) is a monoterpenoid phytochemical that inhibits biofilm formation by proliferating bacterial membrane and causing leakage to important bacterial cells (Beheshti-Rouy et al., 2015)

Extracts of *Camellia sinensis* were found to consists of saponins, tannins, catechin and epigallocatechin gallate that inhibited microorganisms such as *S. mutans, S. salivarius* and *E. coli* and promoting bacterial acid resistance (Rasheed and Haider, 1998).

The crude extracts of *Caesalpinia ferrea martius* fruit were experimented and revealed to have antimicrobial activity such as anthraquinones, alkaloids, depsides, depsidones, flavonoids, lactones, saponins, sugars, tannins, sesquiterpenes and triterpenes. The polyphenols and methoxylated compounds extracted from the fruit showed strong anti-glucosyltransferase activity that could inhibit the growth of cariogenic bacteria; *Candida albicans, Streptococcus mutans, Streptococcus salivarius, Streptococcus oralis* and *Lactobacillus casei* (Sampaio et al., 2009). Even though Streptococcus mutans have been stated to be the main causative agent of dental caries, Streptococcus salivarius tend to produce higher amounts of extracellular polymers that create a suitable habitat for other pathogens to exist (Marsh, 2005). Therefore inhibiting *S. salivarius* is important in disruption of biofilm formation. However, the presence of the tannins in the extract distorted the binding potential of the salivary proteins onto the tooth enamel (Sampaio et al., 2009).

Ziziphus jujube leaves extract has been suggested as an anti-caries agent because of its antimicrobial activity against *S. mutans*. Ziziphus jujuba mill *(Rhanaceae)* commonly located in Southern Asia was found to inhibit cariogenic bacteria due to its antioxidant polyphenols (quercetin, catechin and gallocatechin). The methanol and water extracts disrupted the biofilm formation in a dose-dependent manner that resulted in the best inhibitory mechanism (Damiano et al., 2017).

Shunya Oka et al's *in vitro* experiment on brown algae (Kelp) showed that the macroalgae which is a sulphated polysaccharide inhibited the adhesion of S. mutans onto the enamel. The results clearly indicated the strong antimicrobial activity of Fucoidans in Kelp in the reduction of the presence of oral bacteria. The antimicrobial activity of the Fucoidans also has an effect in the dissolution of water-insoluble glucans (Oka et al., 2020).

4.2 Research Directions and Challenges

The use of natural actives in dentistry to protect the enamel seems to be gaining popularity and becoming more promising. However, the process of incorporating natural actives into dentifrices formulation is quite challenging. One of the main challenges is the stability and phase separation of hydrophobic natural products. There is a difficulty in formulating natural products into aqueous substances because most bioactive compounds are highly volatile and water-insoluble is a major problem (Jeon et al., 2011). Other bioactive compounds are chemically unstable. They tend to deteriorate upon exposure to light, humidity, heat, and oxygen causing undesirable formulations and non-compliance (Turek and Stintzing, 2013). Some phytochemicals also tend to have sour taste which means they must be mixed with a lot of flavours and sweeteners before achieving a satisfying result (Philip et al., 2019).

The process of identifying their chemical components is also challenging. Purification of the crude natural extracts into their specific chemical components to be used in dentistry or drug discovery is stressful. This involves several time-consuming purification and bioassay procedures. There is limited availability of chemically characterised natural supplies to separate the raw products into pure bioactive molecules (Jeon et al., 2011)

Another challenging factor is the retention time of natural actives applied into the oral cavity. To achieve maximum demineralisation-remineralisation process, the oral cavity must be exposed to adequate concentrations of natural actives to disrupt the aetiological pathways of dental biofilms (Philip et al., 2019).

The effect of geographical locations, biodiversity variations, unfavourable seasons and environmental conditions may also affect the growth and supply of natural products that are dominant in specific continents (Jeon et al., 2011). For example, there are different varieties of Propolis mainly found in Brazil. These may affect the bioactivity, traceability, and reproducibility of the honeybees. To account for consistency, traceability and reproducibility, the sources of natural extracts should be properly documented.

Lastly, a challenging factor is knowing the safety of the phytochemical. A lot of food-derived phytochemicals are not expected to be toxic and therefore has been categorised as GRAS (generally recognised as safe) compounds (Freires et al., 2015, Bakkali et al., 2008). However, this does not guarantee the safety of all phytochemicals. For example, the discontinuation with using sanguinarine after its alleged oral leucoplakia linkage (Vlachojannis et al., 2012). However, in 2003, the US Food and Dugs Administration (US FDA) Subcommittee on Oral Health Care Drug Product for Over-the-Counter Human Use stated that the ingredient was safe for use (Vlachojannis et al., 2012).

4.3 Future Work and Recommendations

Addition of natural products to oral care regimens is less costly with reduced side effects (Chen et al., 2020).. It is seen to be sustainable and eco-friendly. Even though natural products have been researched and stated as possessing antimicrobial properties against several ailments including oral health problems, there is still little information on their safety, quality, and interactions with other medications (Groppo et al., 2008). Most of the studies carried by researchers to evaluate the anticaries effect of natural products are *in vitro* analysis (Philip et al., 2019). Extensive *in vivo* and clinical trial studies in the areas of quality, safety, and toxicity to ascertain the long-term exposure to humans is required. Also, further research to determine the actual mechanisms of plaque inhibition on the enamel and the appropriate dosage forms in oral care products is required.

Additionally, the demand to discover new phytochemicals that protect the enamel by inhibiting the activities of cariogenic bacteria is on the rise, making the work of researchers a never-ending process.

Nebu Philip et al suggested that for maximum broad-spectrum effect of anticaries properties, a cross-disciplinary approach of natural products should be evaluated. Further studies on the anticaries ability of natural products in combination with other preventive agents such as chlorhexidine or fluoride should be clinically examined through both *in vitro* and *in vivo* studies (Philip et al., 2019).

Below is a simplified process to consider that may help to minimise the complexities of evaluating natural products for cariostatic benefits (Jeon et al., 2011):

> ➢ Purification process and the source of collection should be reliable and reproducible

> ➢ Hiring of a professional in the field of taxonomy, medicinal and analytical chemistry should be considered

- Extracts of plants intended to be used in formulations should be chemically standardised and characterised before its evaluation
- The process of assessing bioactive sources should be practical and clinically approved. This process involves six steps:

-Finding the natural extracts

-Process of characterising the bioactive sources such as identifying and isolating

-Biological activity of extracts should be validated

-Studies of their toxicity should be carried out

-Regulation processes to ascertain natural extract's safety and efficacy must be followed

CHAPTER FIVE: IMPACT OF FINDINGS AND CONCLUSION

The use of bioactive components of natural extracts have been of increasing interest in recent years as they are a valuable source of oral antimicrobial agents that exhibit minimal toxicity. However, they remain largely unexplored as literature is limited with regards to data on the safety, quality, and efficiency of natural products for use in dentistry. New available technologies make the research and development of antiplaque agents in bioactive molecules accessible and less time consuming.

Technologies such as screening, isolation, and separation of bioactive extracts to reproduce and optimise sources are advancing biosynthetic chemistry and metabolic engineering research.

Well established characterisation and standardisation techniques of natural products are essential cross-disciplinary approaches for future research on cariostatic agents.

Natural products have been researched to be efficacious when used singly or in combination with other preventive agents to provide a synergistic effect. The use of natural products in combination with fluoride in its usual concentrations could provide an enhanced anticaries effect for a stronger enamel.

This review aimed to explore biological active sources of marine and plant extracts that protect the enamel through their antimicrobial activity against cariogenic bacteria. The results indicated that bioactive compounds of natural products inhibit the pathways of cariogenic bacteria by weakening their bacterial cell membrane, disrupt the adhesion of oral microorganisms to the enamel and interfere with the activities of GTF.

From this review, it will be concluded that natural products are important for the development of anticaries agents because they prevent demineralisation and control the incidence of dental caries to promote a stronger tooth structure.

REFERENCES

1. AJAGANNANAVAR, S. L., BATTUR, H., SHAMARAO, S., SIVAKUMAR, V., PATIL, P. U. & SHANAVAS, P. 2014. Effect of aqueous and alcoholic licorice (glycyrrhiza glabra) root extract against streptococcus mutans and lactobacillus acidophilus in comparison to chlorhexidine: an in vitro study. *Journal of international oral health: JIOH,* 6, 29.
2. AL-OTAIBI, M., AL-HARTHY, M., SODER, B., GUSTAFSSON, A. & ANGMAR-MANSSON, B. 2003. Comparative effect of chewing sticks and toothbrushing on plaque removal and gingival health. *Oral health and preventive dentistry,* 1, 301-308.
3. BADET, C. & QUERO, F. 2011. The in vitro effect of manuka honeys on growth and adherence of oral bacteria. *Anaerobe,* 17, 19-22.
4. BAGRAMIAN, R. A., GARCIA-GODOY, F. & VOLPE, A. R. 2009. The global increase in dental caries. A pending public health crisis. *Am J dent,* 22, 3-8.
5. BAKKALI, F., AVERBECK, S., AVERBECK, D. & IDAOMAR, M. 2008. Biological effects of essential oils–a review. *Food and chemical toxicology,* 46, 446-475.
6. BEHESHTI-ROUY, M., AZARSINA, M., REZAIE-SOUFI, L., ALIKHANI, M. Y., ROSHANAIE, G. & KOMAKI, S. 2015. The antibacterial effect of sage extract (Salvia officinalis) mouthwash against Streptococcus mutans in dental plaque: a randomized clinical trial. *Iranian journal of microbiology,* 7, 173.
7. BHAT, N., BAPAT, S., ASAWA, K., TAK, M., CHATURVEDI, P., GUPTA, V. V. & GEORGE, P. P. 2015. The antiplaque efficacy of propolis-based herbal toothpaste: A crossover clinical study. *Journal of natural science, biology, and medicine,* 6, 364.
8. BONESVOLL, P. & GJERMO, P. 1978. A comparison between chlorhexidine and some quaternary ammonium compounds with regard to retention, salivary concentration and plaque-inhibiting effect in the human mouth after mouth rinses. *Archives of oral biology,* 23, 289-294.
9. BORA, A., GOSWAMI, A., KUNDU, G. K. & GHOSH, B. 2014. Antimicrobial efficacy of few commercially available herbal and non-herbal toothpastes against clinically isolated human cariogenic pathogens. *JNDA,* 14, 35-40.
10. BUSSCHER, H. J., ENGELS, E., DIJKSTRA, R. J. & VAN DER MEI, H. C. 2008. Influence of a chitosan on oral bacterial adhesion and growth in vitro. *European Journal of Oral Sciences,* 116, 493-495.
11. CHEN, X., DALIRI, E. B.-M., KIM, N., KIM, J.-R., YOO, D. & OH, D.-H. 2020. Microbial etiology and prevention of dental caries: exploiting natural products to inhibit cariogenic biofilms. *Pathogens,* 9, 569.
12. CHINOU, I. 2008. Primary and secondary metabolites and their biological activity. *CHROMATOGRAPHIC SCIENCE SERIES,* 99, 59.
13. COWAN, M. M. 1999. Plant products as antimicrobial agents. *Clinical microbiology reviews,* 12, 564-582.
14. CURY, J. A. & TENUTA, L. M. A. 2014. Evidence-based recommendation on toothpaste use. *Brazilian oral research,* 28, 1-7.
15. DAMIANO, S., FORINO, M., DE, A., VITALI, L. A., LUPIDI, G. & TAGLIALATELA-SCAFATI, O. 2017. Antioxidant and antibiofilm activities of secondary metabolites from Ziziphus jujuba leaves used for infusion preparation. *Food chemistry,* 230, 24-29.
16. DAVIES, R., ELLWOOD, R. & DAVIES, G. 2003. The rational use of fluoride toothpaste. *International journal of dental hygiene,* 1, 3-8.
17. DE JESUS RAPOSO, M. F., DE MORAIS, A. M. B. & DE MORAIS, R. M. S. C. 2015. Marine polysaccharides from algae with potential biomedical applications. *Marine drugs,* 13, 2967-3028.
18. DEO, P. N. & DESHMUKH, R. 2019. Oral microbiome: Unveiling the fundamentals. *Journal of oral and maxillofacial pathology: JOMFP,* 23, 122.

19. DESBOIS, A. P. & SMITH, V. J. 2010. Antibacterial free fatty acids: activities, mechanisms of action and biotechnological potential. *Applied microbiology and biotechnology,* 85, 1629-1642.
20. DORMAN, H. D. & DEANS, S. G. 2000. Antimicrobial agents from plants: antibacterial activity of plant volatile oils. *Journal of applied microbiology,* 88, 308-316.
21. DREAMSTIME.COM. 2000-2021. *Human tooth structure with description* [Online]. google. [Accessed September 6, 2021 2021].
22. DUARTE, S., GREGOIRE, S., SINGH, A. P., VORSA, N., SCHAICH, K., BOWEN, W. H. & KOO, H. 2006. Inhibitory effects of cranberry polyphenols on formation and acidogenicity of Streptococcus mutans biofilms. *FEMS microbiology letters,* 257, 50-56.
23. DUBEY, N., KUMAR, R. & TRIPATHI, P. 2004. Global promotion of herbal medicine: India's opportunity. *Current science,* 86, 37-41.
24. EMBERY, G., RØLLA, G. & DE L'EUROPE, C. 1992. *Clinical and biological aspects of dentifrices,* Oxford University Press Oxford.
25. FALLER, R. V., EVERSOLE, S. L. & TZEGHAI, G. E. 2011. Enamel protection: a comparison of marketed dentifrice performance against dental erosion. *American Journal of Dentistry,* 24, 205.
26. FEJERSKOV, O., NYVAD, B. & KIDD, E. 2015. *Dental caries: the disease and its clinical management,* John Wiley & Sons.
27. FERRAZZANO, G. F., SCIOSCIA, E., SATERIALE, D., PASTORE, G., COLICCHIO, R., PAGLIUCA, C., CANTILE, T., ALCIDI, B., CODA, M. & INGENITO, A. 2017. In vitro antibacterial activity of pomegranate juice and peel extracts on cariogenic bacteria. *BioMed research international,* 2017.
28. FERREIRA, M. C., RAMOS-JORGE, M. L., DELBEM, A. C. B. & DE SOUSA VIEIRAC, R. 2013. Effect of toothpastes with different abrasives on eroded human enamel: An in situ/ex vivo study. *The open dentistry journal,* 7, 132.
29. FRAIHAT, N., MADAE'EN, S., BENCZE, Z., HERCZEG, A. & VARGA, O. 2019. Clinical effectiveness and cost-effectiveness of oral-health promotion in dental caries prevention among children: Systematic review and meta-analysis. *International journal of environmental research and public health,* 16, 2668.
30. FREIRES, I. A., DENNY, C., BENSO, B., DE ALENCAR, S. M. & ROSALEN, P. L. 2015. Antibacterial activity of essential oils and their isolated constituents against cariogenic bacteria: a systematic review. *Molecules,* 20, 7329-7358.
31. GREENWALL, L. H., GREENWALL-COHEN, J. & WILSON, N. H. 2019. Charcoal-containing dentifrices. *British dental journal,* 226, 697-700.
32. GREGOIRE, S., SINGH, A., VORSA, N. & KOO, H. 2007. Influence of cranberry phenolics on glucan synthesis by glucosyltransferases and Streptococcus mutans acidogenicity. *Journal of applied microbiology,* 103, 1960-1968.
33. GROPPO, F. C., BERGAMASCHI, C. D. C., COGO, K., FRANZ-MONTAN, M., MOTTA, R. H. L. & ANDRADE, E. D. D. 2008. Use of phytotherapy in dentistry. *Phytotherapy Research,* 22, 993-998.
34. GROSOFSKY, A., ADKINS, S., BASTHOLM, R., MEYER, L., KRUEGER, L., MEYER, J. & TORMA, P. 2003. Tooth color: effects on judgments of attractiveness and age. *Perceptual and motor skills,* 96, 43-48.
35. HANNAH, J., JOHNSON, J. & KUFTINEC, M. 1989. Long-term clinical evaluation of toothpaste and oral rinse containing sanguinaria extract in controlling plaque, gingival inflammation, and sulcular bleeding during orthodontic treatment. *American Journal of Orthodontics and Dentofacial Orthopedics,* 96, 199-207.
36. HIRASAWA, M., SHOUJI, N., NETA, T., FUKUSHIMA, K. & TAKADA, K. 1999. Three kinds of antibacterial substances from Lentinus edodes (Berk.) Sing.(Shiitake, an edible mushroom). *International Journal of Antimicrobial Agents,* 11, 151-157.

37. HORNER, C., MAWER, D. & WILCOX, M. 2012. Reduced susceptibility to chlorhexidine in staphylococci: is it increasing and does it matter? *Journal of antimicrobial chemotherapy,* 67, 2547-2559.
38. HOSSEINI TAFRESHI, A. & SHARIATI, M. 2009. Dunaliella biotechnology: methods and applications. *Journal of applied microbiology,* 107, 14-35.
39. ISLAM, B., KHAN, S. N., HAQUE, I., ALAM, M., MUSHFIQ, M. & KHAN, A. U. 2008. Novel anti-adherence activity of mulberry leaves: inhibition of Streptococcus mutans biofilm by 1-deoxynojirimycin isolated from Morus alba. *Journal of antimicrobial chemotherapy,* 62, 751-757.
40. JAFARI, S., MOBASHER, M. A., NAJAFIPOUR, S., GHASEMI, Y., MOHKAM, M., EBRAHIMI, M. A. & MOBASHER, N. 2018. Antibacterial potential of Chlorella vulgaris and Dunaliella salina extracts against Streptococcus mutans. *Jundishapur Journal of Natural Pharmaceutical Products,* 13.
41. JEON, J.-G., ROSALEN, P., FALSETTA, M. & KOO, H. 2011. Natural products in caries research: current (limited) knowledge, challenges and future perspective. *Caries research,* 45, 243-263.
42. JOHNSON, N. & BAIN, C. 2000. Tobacco and oral disease. *British Dental Journal,* 189, 200-206.
43. JONES, F. 2001. Teeth and bones: applications of surface science to dental materials and related biomaterials. *Surface science reports,* 42, 75-205.
44. JUN, J.-Y., JUNG, M.-J., JEONG, I.-H., YAMAZAKI, K., KAWAI, Y. & KIM, B.-M. 2018. Antimicrobial and antibiofilm activities of sulfated polysaccharides from marine algae against dental plaque bacteria. *Marine drugs,* 16, 301.
45. KANDALE, A., MEENA, A., RAO, M., PANDA, P., MANGAL, A., REDDY, G. & BABU, R. 2011. Marine algae: an introduction, food value and medicinal uses. *Journal of Pharmacy Research,* 4, 219-221.
46. KIDD AND JOYSTON-BECHAL. 1997. *Diagram of the caries process as regular fl ux of demineralisation (destruction) and remineralisation (repair)* [Online]. Scientific Figure on ResearchGate.: /www.researchgate.net/figure/Diagram-of-the-caries-process-as-regular-fl-ux-of-demineralisation-destruction-and_fig2_6591922 [accessed 6 Sep, 2021]. [Accessed September 6, 2021 2021].
47. KIM, Y.-H., KIM, J. H., JIN, H.-J. & LEE, S. Y. 2013. Antimicrobial activity of ethanol extracts of Laminaria japonica against oral microorganisms. *Anaerobe,* 21, 34-38.
48. KLEINBERG, I. 2002. A mixed-bacteria ecological approach to understanding the role of the oral bacteria in dental caries causation: an alternative to Streptococcus mutans and the specific-plaque hypothesis. *Critical Reviews in Oral Biology & Medicine,* 13, 108-125.
49. KOO, H., ROSALEN, P. L., CURY, J. A., PARK, Y. K. & BOWEN, W. H. 2002. Effects of compounds found in propolis on Streptococcus mutans growth and on glucosyltransferase activity. *Antimicrobial agents and chemotherapy,* 46, 1302-1309.
50. KRISHNA, M., YORK, M., CHIN, T., GNANAKUMARAN, G., HESLEGRAVE, J., DERBRIDGE, C., HUISSOON, A., DIWAKAR, L., EREN, E. & CROSSMAN, R. 2014. Multi-centre retrospective analysis of anaphylaxis during general anaesthesia in the U nited K ingdom: aetiology and diagnostic performance of acute serum tryptase. *Clinical & Experimental Immunology,* 178, 399-404.
51. LAROCHE, M., BERGERON, J. & BARBARO-FORLEO, G. 2001. Targeting consumers who are willing to pay more for environmentally friendly products. *Journal of consumer marketing.*
52. LEE, Y.-C., CHO, S.-G., KIM, S.-W. & KIM, J. N. 2019. Anticariogenic potential of korean native plant extracts against Streptococcus mutans. *Planta medica,* 85, 1242-1252.
53. LENANDER-LUMIKARI, M. & LOIMARANTA, V. 2000. Saliva and dental caries. *Advances in dental research,* 14, 40-47.

54. LI, X., WANG, J., JOINER, A. & CHANG, J. 2014. The remineralisation of enamel: a review of the literature. *Journal of dentistry,* 42, S12-S20.
55. LUTOVAC, M., POPOVA, O. V., MACANOVIC, G., KRISTINA, R., LUTOVAC, B., KETIN, S. & BIOCANIN, R. 2017. Testing the effect of aggressive beverage on the damage of enamel structure. *Open access Macedonian journal of medical sciences,* 5, 987.
56. MARINHO, V. C., CHONG, L. Y., WORTHINGTON, H. V. & WALSH, T. 2016. Fluoride mouthrinses for preventing dental caries in children and adolescents. *Cochrane database of systematic reviews.*
57. MARSH, P. D. 2005. Dental plaque: biological significance of a biofilm and community life-style. *Journal of clinical periodontology,* 32, 7-15.
58. MARTINS, M. L., DE FRANÇA LEITE, K. L., PACHECO-FILHO, E. F., DE MIRANDA PEREIRA, A. F., ROMANOS, M. T. V., MAIA, L. C., FONSECA-GONÇALVES, A., PADILHA, W. W. N. & CAVALCANTI, Y. W. 2018. Efficacy of red propolis hydro-alcoholic extract in controlling Streptococcus mutans biofilm build-up and dental enamel demineralization. *Archives of oral biology,* 93, 56-65.
59. MOREIRA, M. R., SOUZA, A. B., SOARES, S., BIANCHI, T. C., DE SOUZA EUGÊNIO, D., LEMES, D. C., MARTINS, C. H. G., DA SILVA MORAES, T., TAVARES, D. C. & FERREIRA, N. H. 2016. ent-Kaurenoic acid-rich extract from Mikania glomerata: In vitro activity against bacteria responsible for dental caries. *Fitoterapia,* 112, 211-216.
60. MORGAN, A. 2008. Vital guide to Preventing dental caries. *Vital,* 5, 21-24.
61. NEWBRUN, E. 1982. Sugar and dental caries: a review of human studies. *Science,* 217, 418-423.
62. NOSTRO, A., CANNATELLI, M., CRISAFI, G., MUSOLINO, A., PROCOPIO, F. & ALONZO, V. 2004. Modifications of hydrophobicity, in vitro adherence and cellular aggregation of Streptococcus mutans by Helichrysum italicum extract. *Letters in applied microbiology,* 38, 423-427.
63. OKA, S., OKABE, M., TSUBURA, S., MIKAMI, M. & IMAI, A. 2020. Properties of fucoidans beneficial to oral healthcare. *Odontology,* 108, 34-42.
64. OSUJP, O., LEAKE, J., CHIPMAN, M., NIKIFORUK, G., LOCKER, D. & LEVINE, N. 1988. Risk factors for dental fluorosis in a fluoridated community. *Journal of dental research,* 67, 1488-1492.
65. PACEY, L. 2012. Is seaweed superior to toothpaste? *British Dental Journal,* 213.
66. PAGLIARULO, C., DE VITO, V., PICARIELLO, G., COLICCHIO, R., PASTORE, G., SALVATORE, P. & VOLPE, M. G. 2016. Inhibitory effect of pomegranate (Punica granatum l.) polyphenol extracts on the bacterial growth and survival of clinical isolates of pathogenic Staphylococcus aureus and Escherichia coli. *Food chemistry,* 190, 824-831.
67. PAI, M. R., ACHARYA, L. D. & UDUPA, N. 2004. Evaluation of antiplaque activity of Azadirachta indica leaf extract gel—a 6-week clinical study. *Journal of ethnopharmacology,* 90, 99-103.
68. PEMBERTON, M. & GIBSON, J. 2012. Chlorhexidine and hypersensitivity reactions in dentistry. *British dental journal,* 213, 547-550.
69. PHILIP, N., LEISHMAN, S. & WALSH, L. 2019. Potential role for natural products in dental caries control. *Oral Health Prev. Dent,* 17, 479-485.
70. POURESLAMI, H. R., MAKAREM, A. & MOJAB, F. 2008. Paraclinical effects of miswak extract on dental plaque. *Dental Research Journal,* 4, 106-110.
71. PRABAKAR, J., JOHN, J., ARUMUGHAM, M. & KUMAR, P. 2019. Go natural, say no to chemicals—A systematic review on effectiveness of green tea extract containing formulations on dental caries. *Asian J Pharm Clin Res,* 12, 63-69.
72. PRASANTH, M. & RATHA, S. N. 2014. Antimicrobial Property of Herbal Toothpastes: An In-Vitro Analysis. *Research Journal of Pharmacology and Pharmacodynamics,* 6, 30-35.

73. RASHEED, A. & HAIDER, M. 1998. Antibacterial activity of Camellia sinensis extracts against dental caries. *Archives of pharmacal research,* 21, 348-352.
74. RASOOLI, I., SHAYEGH, S. & ASTANEH, S. D. A. 2009. The effect of Mentha spicata and Eucalyptus camaldulensis essential oils on dental biofilm. *International journal of dental hygiene,* 7, 196-203.
75. SAMPAIO, F. C., MARIA DO SOCORRO, V. P., DIAS, C. S., COSTA, V. C. O., CONDE, N. C. & BUZALAF, M. A. 2009. In vitro antimicrobial activity of Caesalpinia ferrea Martius fruits against oral pathogens. *Journal of ethnopharmacology,* 124, 289-294.
76. SEAL, M., RISHI, R., SATISH, G., DIVYA, K., TALUKDAR, P. & MANIYAR, R. 2016. Herbal panacea: The need for today in dentistry. *Journal of International Society of Preventive & Community Dentistry,* 6, 105.
77. SEDIGHINIA, F. & AFSHAR, A. S. 2012. Antibacterial activity of Glycyrrhiza glabra against oral pathogens: an in vitro study. *Avicenna journal of phytomedicine,* 2, 118.
78. SELWITZ, R. H., ISMAIL, A. I. & PITTS, N. B. 2007. Dental caries. *The Lancet,* 369, 51-59.
79. SHEIHAM, A. 2005. Oral health, general health and quality of life. SciELO Public Health.
80. SHINADA, K., TAGASHIRA, M., WATANABE, H., SOPAPORNAMORN, P., KANAYAMA, A., KANDA, T., IKEDA, M. & KAWAGUCHI, Y. 2007. Hop bract polyphenols reduced three-day dental plaque regrowth. *Journal of dental research,* 86, 848-851.
81. SINGER, A. C., CROWLEY, D. E. & THOMPSON, I. P. 2003. Secondary plant metabolites in phytoremediation and biotransformation. *TRENDS in Biotechnology,* 21, 123-130.
82. SKABA, D., MORAWIEC, T., TANASIEWICZ, M., MERTAS, A., BOBELA, E., SZLISZKA, E., SKUCHA-NOWAK, M., DAWIEC, M., YAMAMOTO, R. & ISHIAI, S. 2013. Influence of the toothpaste with brazilian ethanol extract propolis on the oral cavity health. *Evidence-Based Complementary and Alternative Medicine,* 2013.
83. STAMM, J. W. 2007. Multi-function toothpastes for better oral health: a behavioural perspective. *International Dental Journal,* 57, 351-363.
84. SUBRAMANIAM, P., DWIVEDI, S., UMA, E. & BABU, K. G. 2012. Effect of pomegranate and aloe vera extract on streptococcus mutans: An in vitro study. *Dental Hypotheses,* 3, 99.
85. SUJATHA, L., GOVARDHAN, T. L. & RANGAIAH, G. S. 2012. Antibacterial activity of green seaweeds on oral bacteria.
86. SWAMY, M. A. 2011. Marine algal sources for treating bacterial diseases. *Advances in food and nutrition research,* 64, 71-84.
87. TAHMASSEBI, J., DUGGAL, M., MALIK-KOTRU, G. & CURZON, M. 2006. Soft drinks and dental health: a review of the current literature. *Journal of dentistry,* 34, 2-11.
88. TAKAHASHI, N. & NYVAD, B. 2010. The Role of Bacteria in the Caries Process: Ecological Perspectives. *Journal of Dental Research,* 90, 294-303.
89. TEANPAISAN, R., KAWSUD, P., PAHUMUNTO, N. & PURIPATTANAVONG, J. 2017. Screening for antibacterial and antibiofilm activity in Thai medicinal plant extracts against oral microorganisms. *Journal of traditional and complementary medicine,* 7, 172-177.
90. THOMAS, N. V. & KIM, S.-K. 2013. Beneficial effects of marine algal compounds in cosmeceuticals. *Marine drugs,* 11, 146-164.
91. TUREK, C. & STINTZING, F. C. 2013. Stability of essential oils: a review. *Comprehensive reviews in food science and food safety,* 12, 40-53.
92. TWETMAN, S., AXELSSON, S., DAHLGREN, H., HOLM, A. K., KÄLLESTÅL, C., LAGERLÖF, F., LINGSTRÖM, P., MEJÀRE, I., NORDENRAM, G. & NORLUND, A. 2003. Caries-preventive effect of fluoride toothpaste: a systematic review. *Acta Odontologica Scandinavica,* 61, 347-355.
93. VELLAPPALLY, S., FIALA, Z., ŠMEJKALOVÁ, J., JACOB, V., SHRIHARSHA, P., FIALA, Z. & SMEJKALOVÁ, J. 2007. Influence of tobacco use in dental caries development. *Central European journal of public health,* 15.
94. VLACHOJANNIS, C., MAGORA, F. & CHRUBASIK, S. 2012. Rise and fall of oral health products with Canadian bloodroot extract. *Phytotherapy Research,* 26, 1423-1426.

95. WEST, N. X. & JOINER, A. 2014. Enamel mineral loss. *Journal of dentistry,* 42, S2-S11.
96. YADAV, K. & PRAKASH, S. 2017. Dental caries: A microbiological approach. *J Clin Infect Dis Pract,* 2, 1-15.
97. ZHENG, L., OH, S., JEON, J., MOON, B., KWON, H., LIM, S., AN, B. & KANG, C. 2012. The dietary effects of fermented Chlorella vulgaris (CBT®) on production performance, liver lipids and intestinal microflora in laying hens. *Asian-Australasian journal of animal sciences,* 25, 261.

YOUR KNOWLEDGE HAS VALUE

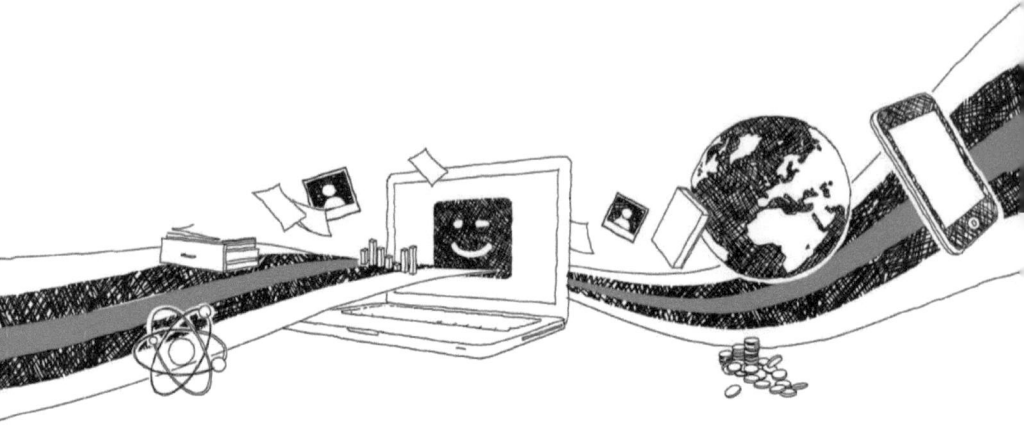

- We will publish your bachelor's and master's thesis, essays and papers

- Your own eBook and book - sold worldwide in all relevant shops

- Earn money with each sale

Upload your text at www.GRIN.com and publish for free

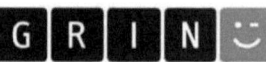